For all who seek healing.

Natural forces within us

are the true healers of disease.

—HIPPOCRATES

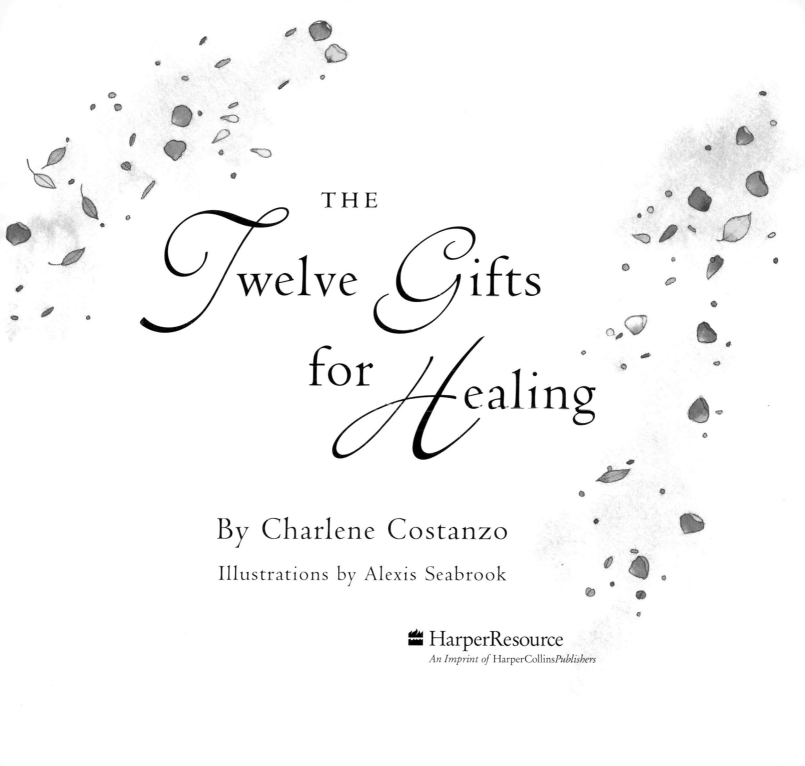

THE

Twelve Gifts
for Healing

By Charlene Costanzo

Illustrations by Alexis Seabrook

HarperResource

An Imprint of HarperCollins*Publishers*

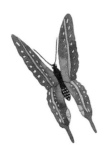

HarperCollins books may be purchased for educational, business, or sales promotional use.
For information please write: Special Markets Department,
HarperCollins Publishers, Inc., 10 East 53rd Street, New York, NY 10022.

FIRST EDITION

PHOTO-TINTING BY RICHARD WAXBERG / DANCING BEARS DESIGN AND TODD MCQUEEN
BOOK DESIGN BY DEBORAH KERNER / DANCING BEARS DESIGN

PHOTO CREDITS: PAGE 17: PHOTODISC / GETTY IMAGES. PAGES 19, 21, 25, 29, 31, 33, 35, 37:
COURTESY OF GETTY IMAGES. PAGE 23: ROBERT GLUSIC / PHOTODISC / GETTY IMAGES.
PAGE 27: COURTESY OF DIGITAL VISION.
PAGE 39: MICHAEL STUCKEY, COMSTOCK IMAGES.

ILLUSTRATIONS COPYRIGHT © 2004 BY ALEXIS SEABROOK

The Library of Congress Cataloging-in-Publication Data has been applied for.

ISBN: 0-06-621128-X

04   05   06   07   08   ❖/ TP   10   9   8   7   6   5   4   3   2   1

There are different kinds of gifts . . .

all from the same Spirit.

Eagerly cultivate the greater gifts . . .

faith, hope, and love.

The greatest of these is love.

—FROM THE FIRST LETTER

TO THE CORINTHIANS

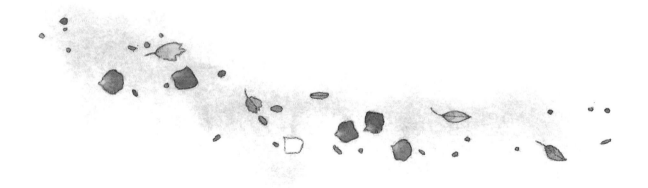

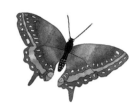

Love heals.

—THE BUDDHA

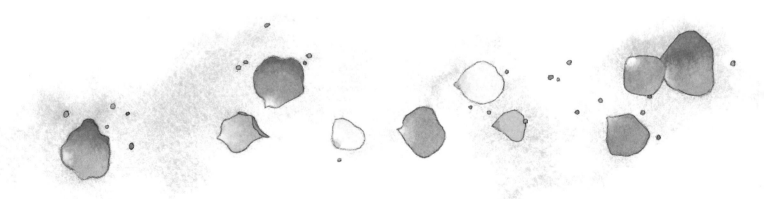

To **Amanda**

From **Mama Klesko**

Because **I love you.** ♡

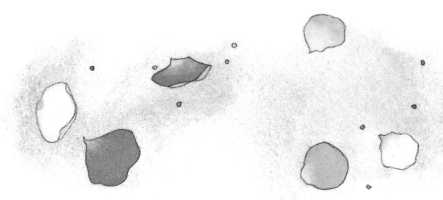
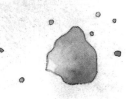

Long ago during a troubled time, an ailing young woman
journeyed to find the old woman who was known as the wise one.
Even though the old woman had never had children of her own,
everyone called her "Mater," which means mother.

When the young woman arrived at the old woman's door, she said,
"Mater, I have heard you know of a healing place.
Will you take me there?"

The old woman was moved by what she saw in the young woman's eyes
and invited her to rest awhile. After sharing a simple meal,
the old woman took the young woman's hands and said,
"Come, daughter. I will show you. Someday, show others."

She led the girl on a tour of the land. In a field they scattered dandelion
seeds with their breath. On a hill they watched clouds take shape and
move across the sky. By the sea they sat where waves could wash
their feet. At each place, the young woman asked,
"Is there healing power here, Mater?"

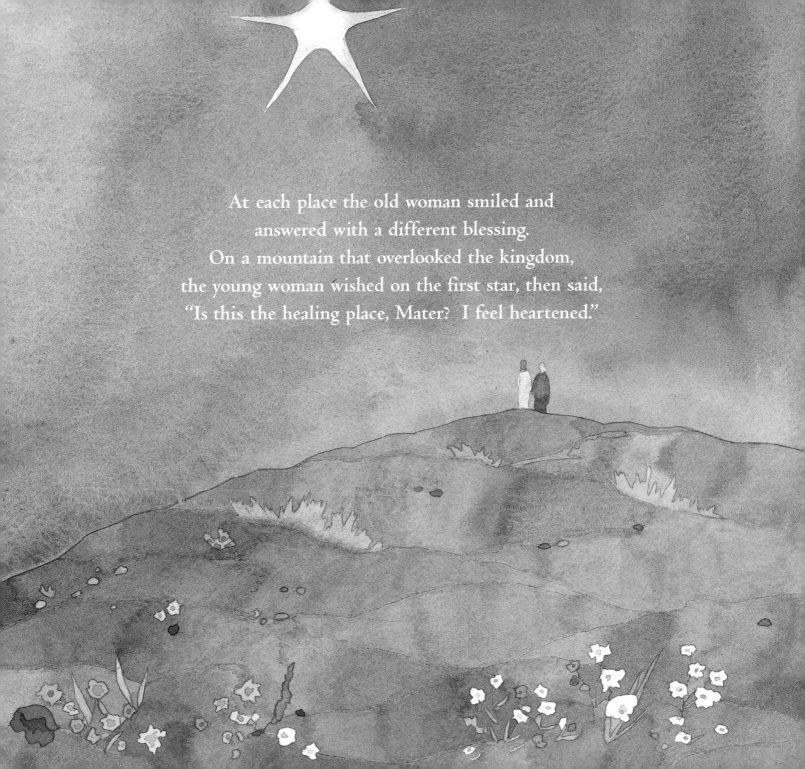

At each place the old woman smiled and
answered with a different blessing.
On a mountain that overlooked the kingdom,
the young woman wished on the first star, then said,
"Is this the healing place, Mater? I feel heartened."

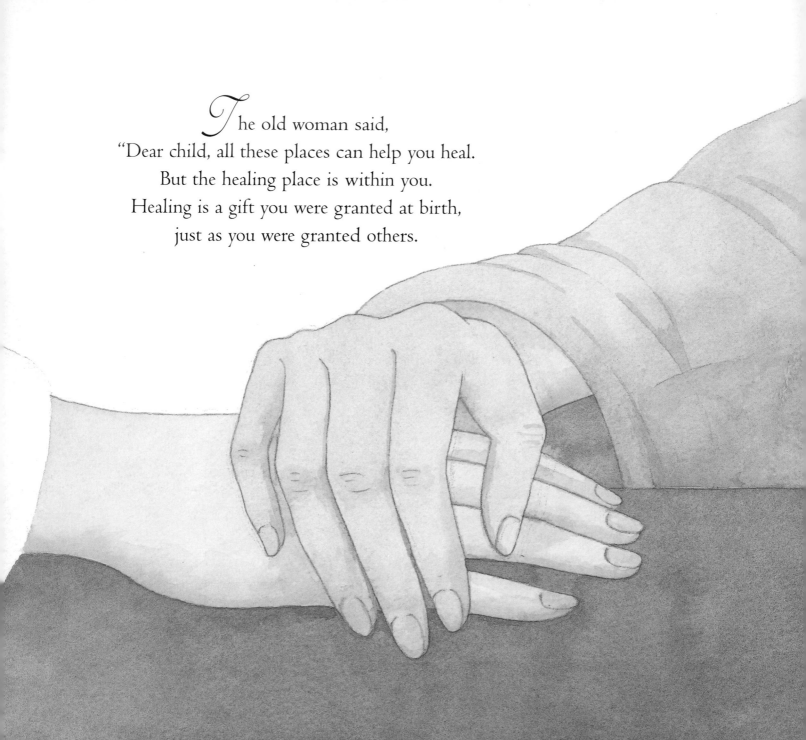

The old woman said,
"Dear child, all these places can help you heal.
But the healing place is within you.
Healing is a gift you were granted at birth,
just as you were granted others.

Use your gifts, child.
Use the beauty, the courage, the hope, and the love that is in you.
Call upon your strength. Use compassion and faith.
Even during sad times joy is within you. Bring it forth.
Wisdom is there to guide you.
Use any one of your gifts and you will rouse
the power of your healing place.
Use all of them and you will sustain it."

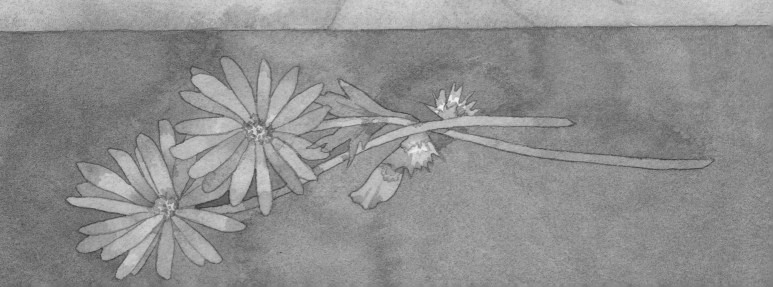

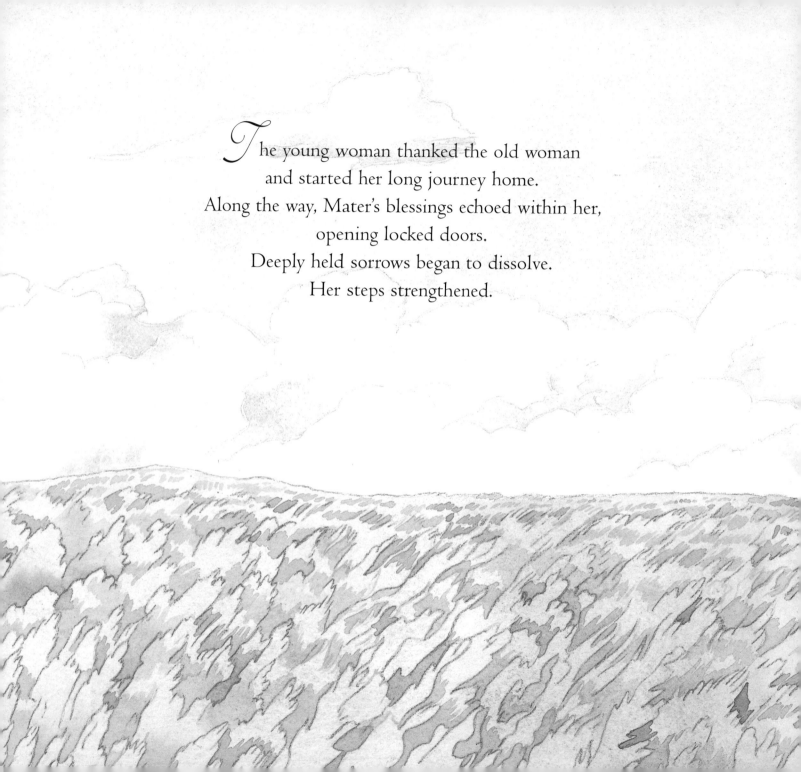

The young woman thanked the old woman
and started her long journey home.
Along the way, Mater's blessings echoed within her,
opening locked doors.
Deeply held sorrows began to dissolve.
Her steps strengthened.

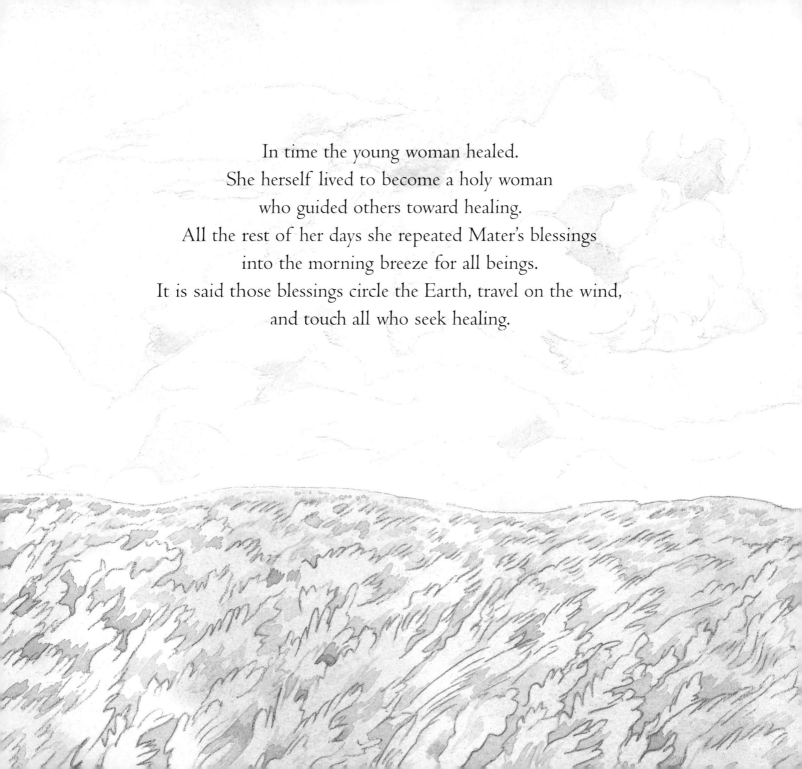

In time the young woman healed.
She herself lived to become a holy woman
who guided others toward healing.
All the rest of her days she repeated Mater's blessings
into the morning breeze for all beings.
It is said those blessings circle the Earth, travel on the wind,
and touch all who seek healing.

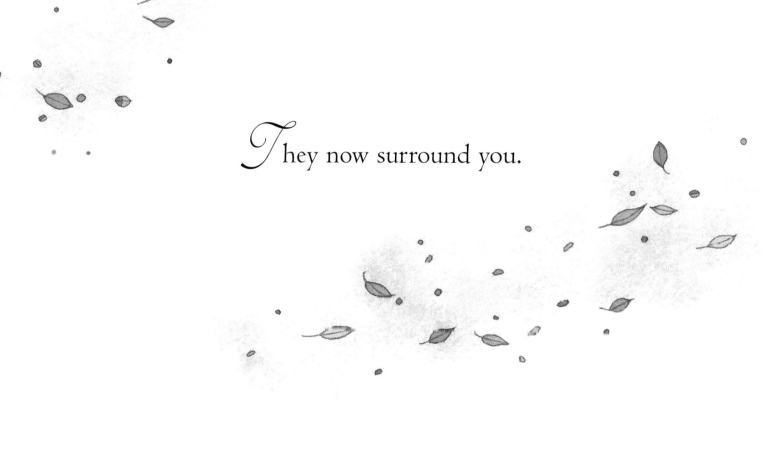

They now surround you.

May you allow fear to soften and melt away.

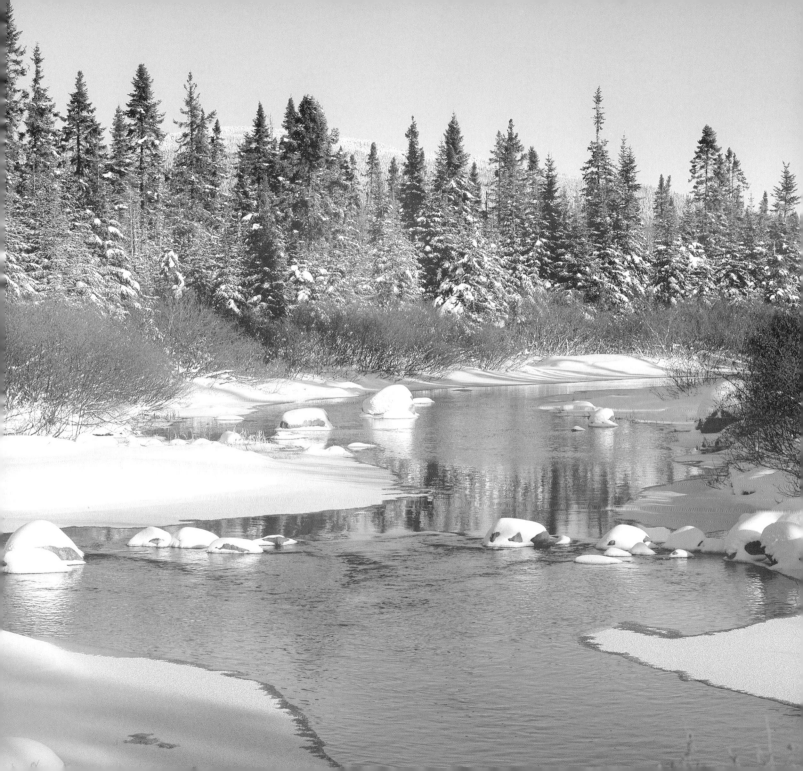

May you release all regrets and resentments.

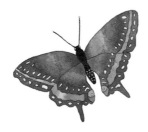

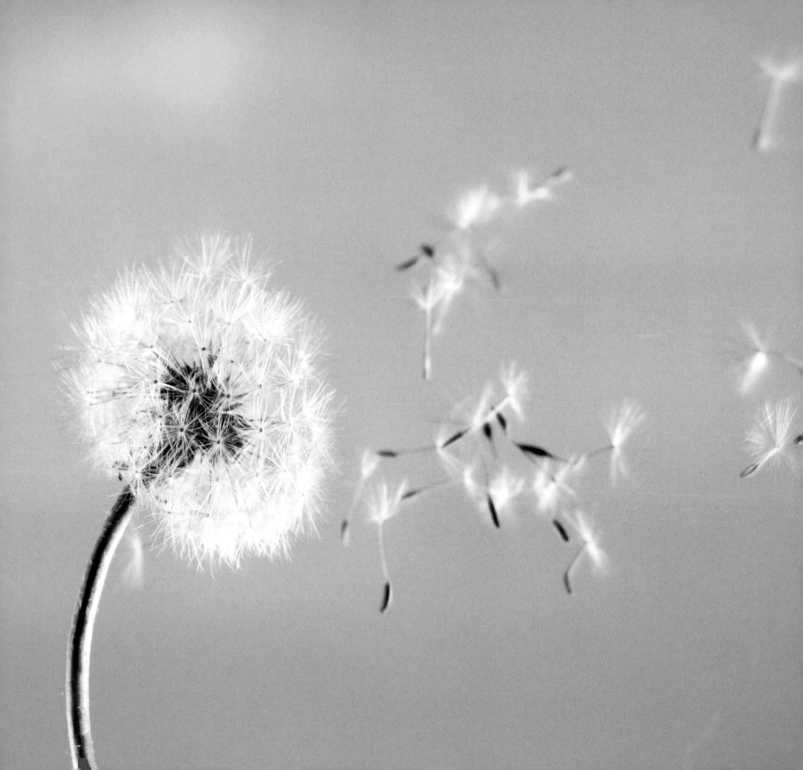

May you see the world with wonder.

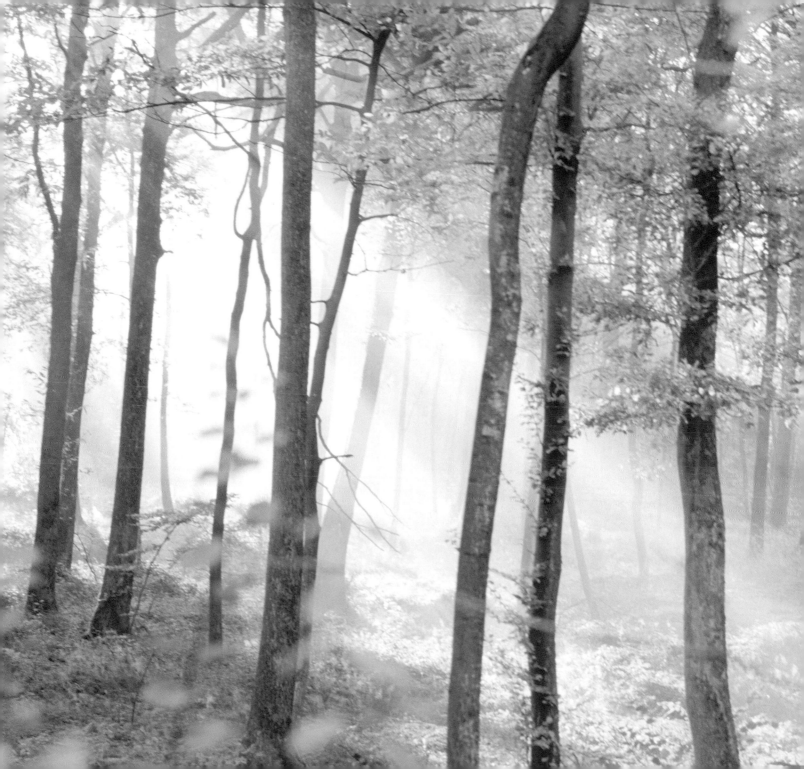

And may you imagine only good things.

May hope rise within you.

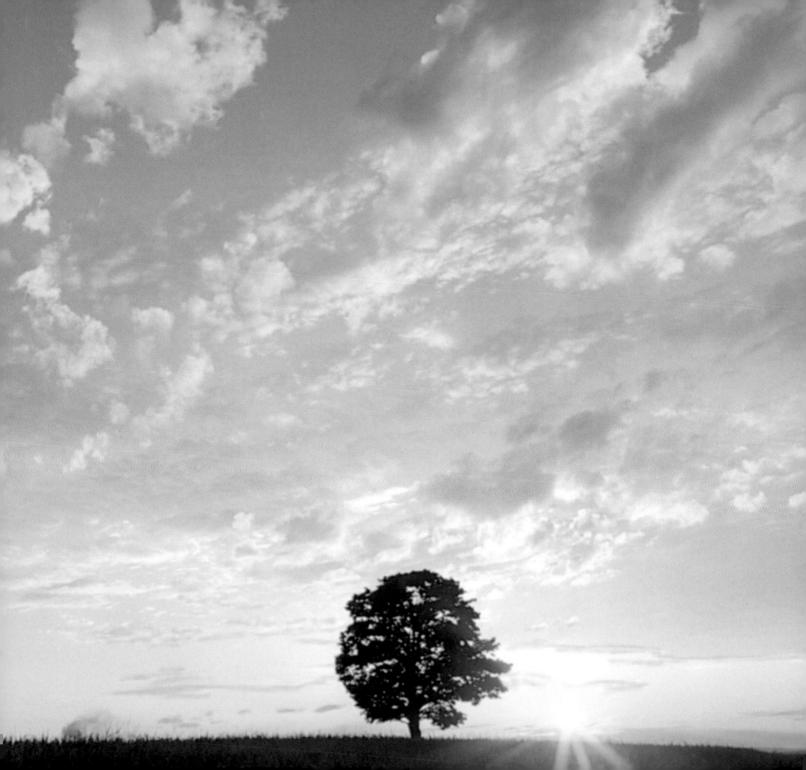

May peace wash over you.

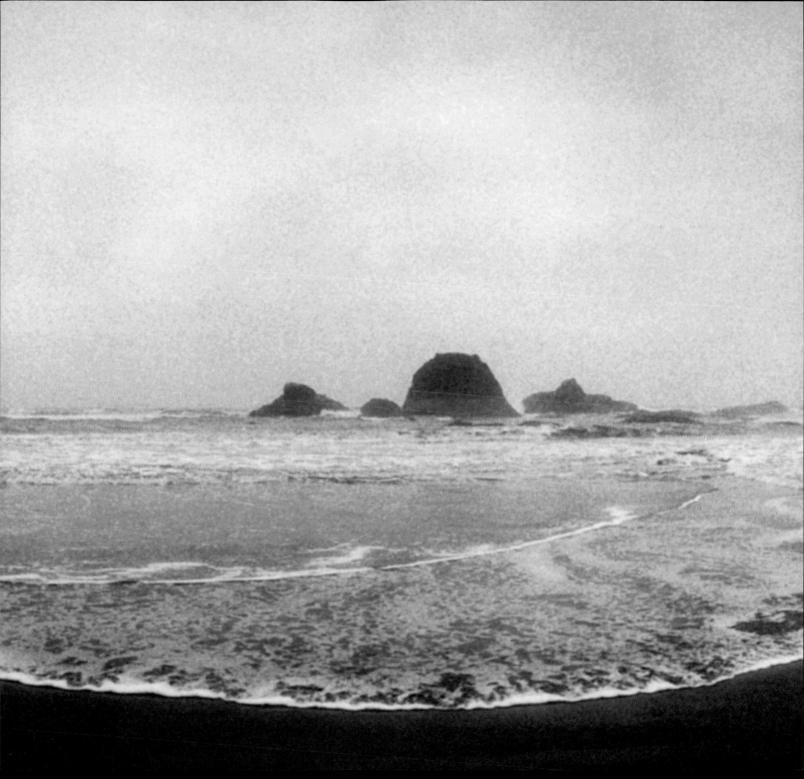

May you hear the voice of wisdom.

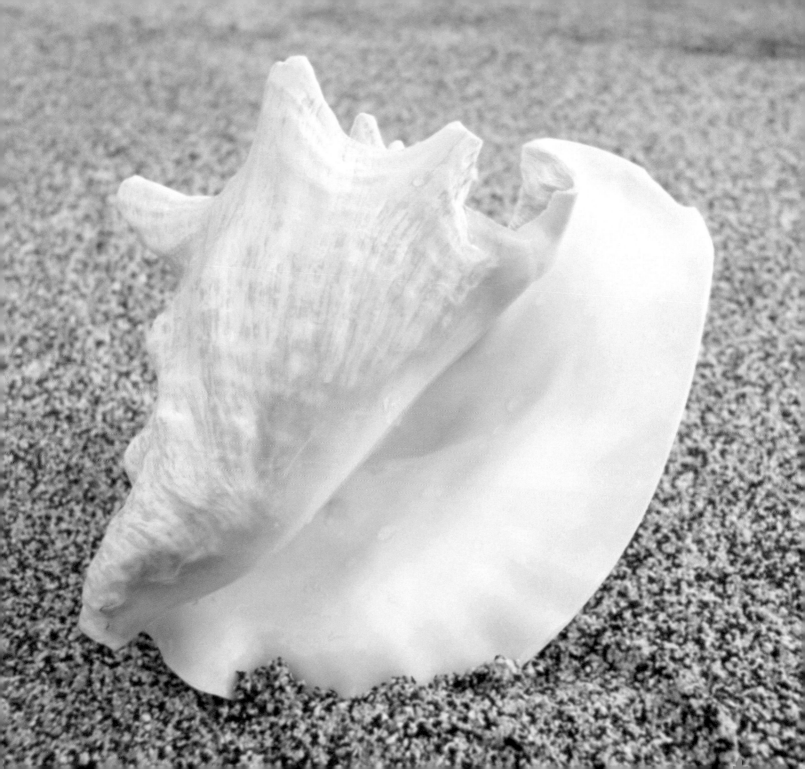

Listening, may you act with trust.

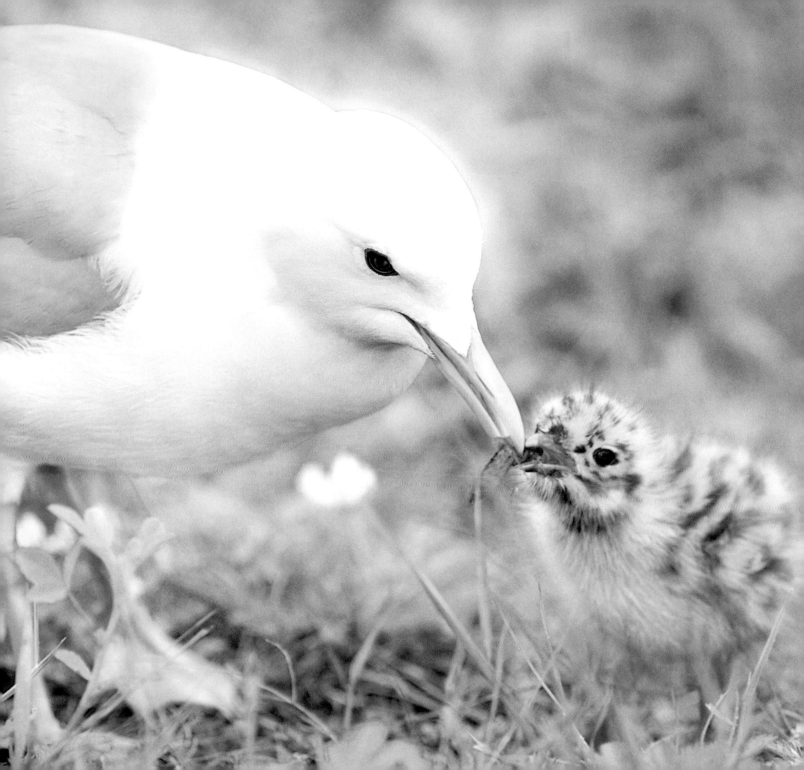

May your heart open.

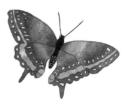

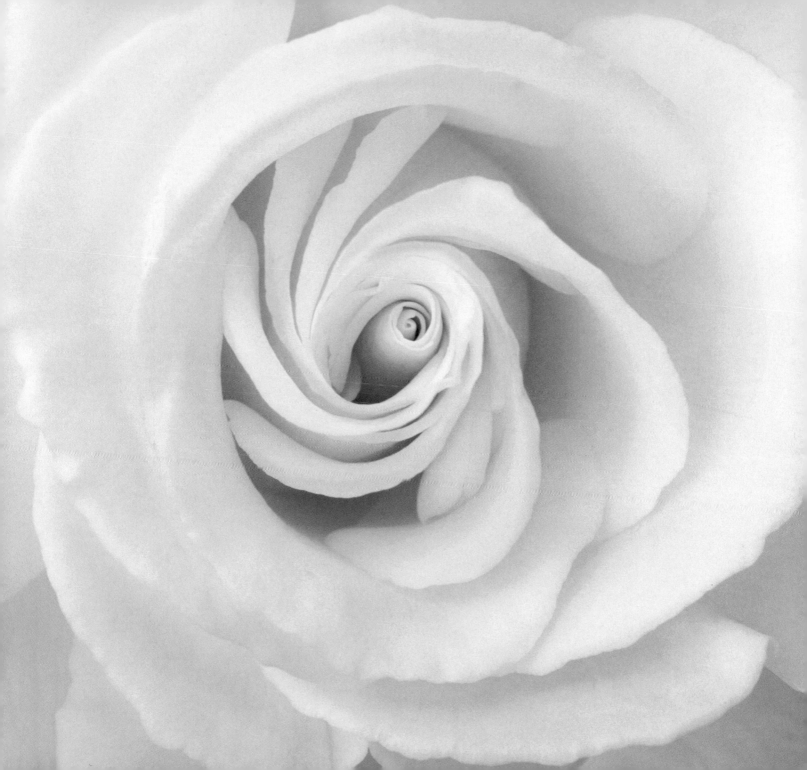

May joy emerge.

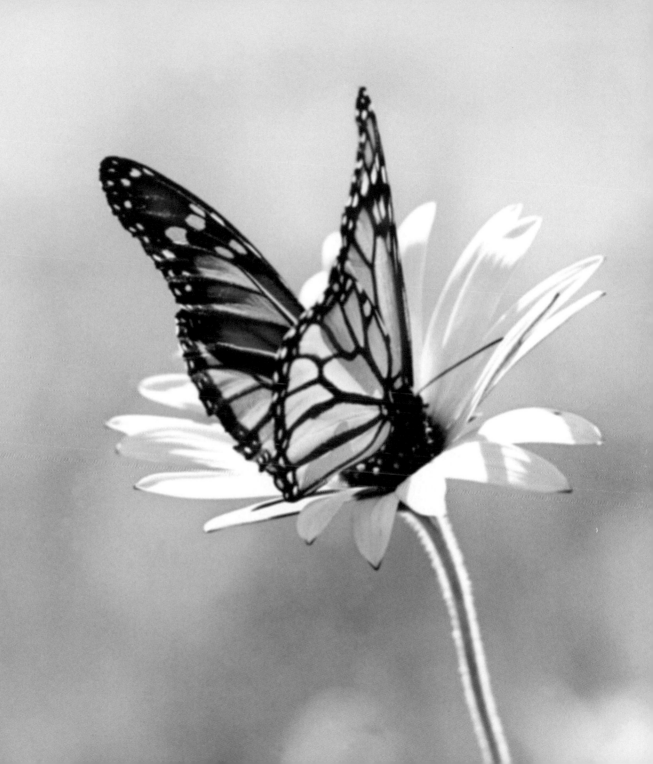

May love flow through you.

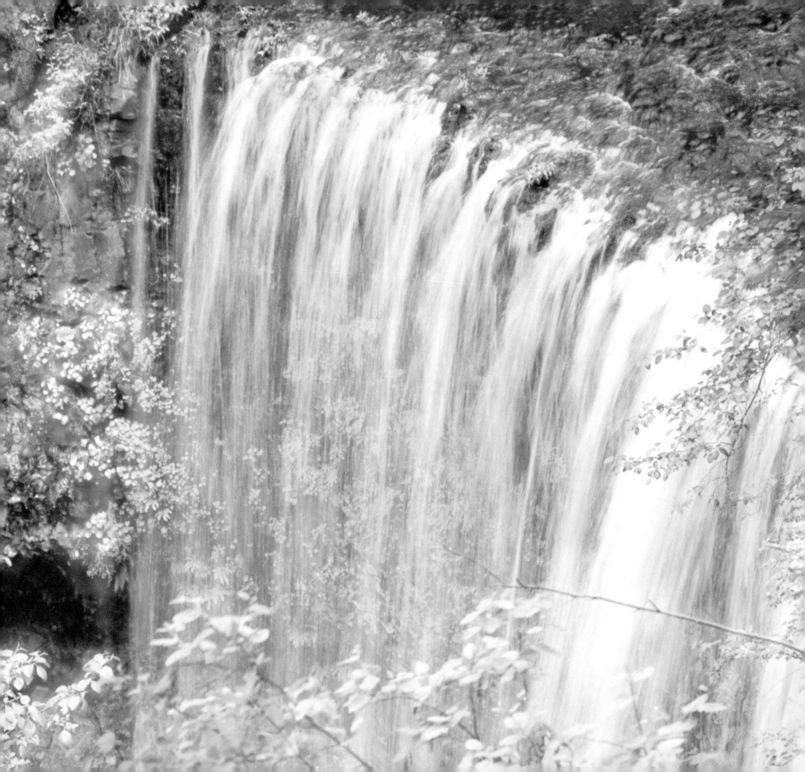

May you heal and help others.

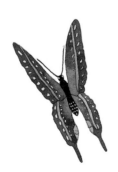

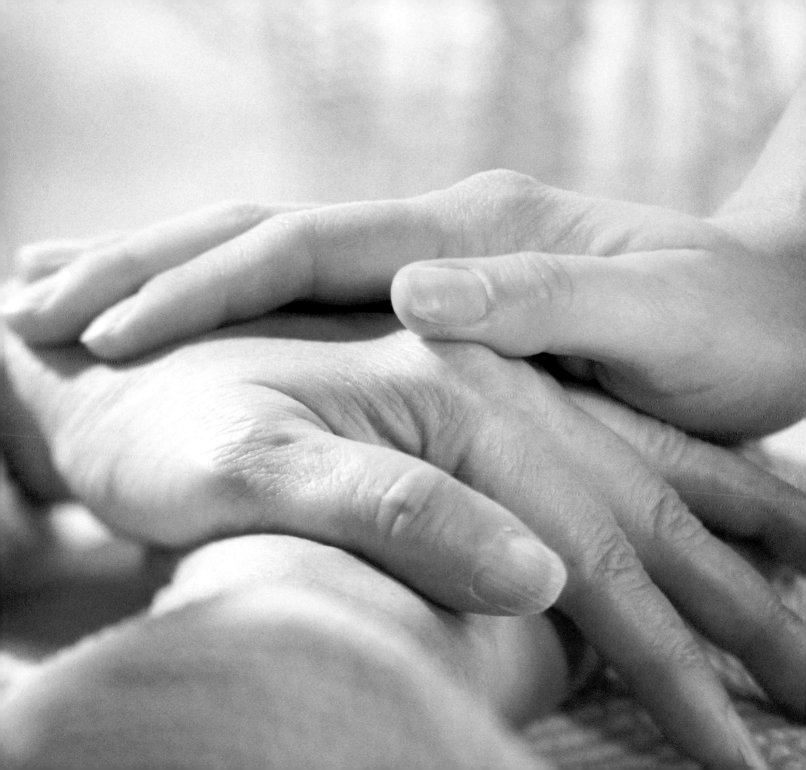

Strive for the greater gifts and

I will show you a still more excellent way.

—I CORINTHIANS 12:31

Afterword

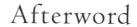

No matter who we are, where we live, what we look like, the circumstances of our birth, or the situations we face, each of us has gifts within us. *Strength, beauty, courage, compassion, hope, joy, talent, imagination, reverence, wisdom, love,* and *faith* are among them. They are not like material presents we unwrap and hold in our hands. We can't see these gifts with our eyes. But they are real and powerful. When we open ourselves to them, they can enrich every aspect of our lives. They can help us transform challenges into opportunities and tragedies into triumphs. They can help us make a difference in the world.

I had come to believe this with all my heart. It is the essence of my first book, *The Twelve Gifts of Birth.* My belief in its message was so strong that it led me, with my husband, to self publish the book, move into a motor home, and travel the country to read the short story in schools, shelters, bookstores, churches, hospitals, and prisons. My belief was reinforced every time I saw resonance in the eyes of those who heard it.

Then one day in Alaska, at the last stop of our tour, I stroked my throat, touched a lump, and felt a chill.

I was diagnosed with two forms of non-Hodgkin's lymphoma, one for which present-day medicine says there is no cure. Although death was not imminent, it seemed close. For several days, I felt frozen with fear, betrayed. I wondered if I would experience peace and joy again.

The disease led me to examine my life, my lifestyle, and my convictions.

Prior to starting chemotherapy, my oncologist said, *"This is a time to call upon strength. Do what makes you strong."*

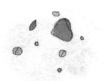

His words caused me to consider what I had written in *The Twelve Gifts of Birth*. About strength I had said, *"May you remember to call upon it whenever you need it."* I had offered that advice to others. Could I heed it now? Was strength fully available to me? Could I summon it? How?

About hope I had written, *"Through each passage and season may you trust the goodness of life."* Could I trust in the midst of this crisis?

While undergoing chemotherapy, I explored many complementary therapies. How might I help my body return to wholeness? I prayed for guidance. This "healing place" story and the twelve blessings in this book were among the answers I received. "Use your gifts," wisdom whispered, "especially *love*." I understood that, besides releasing cancer cells, I needed to heal on other levels. Using love, I needed to release hatred of the aberrant cells. Using compassion, I needed to release regrets and resentments. Using hope, I needed to release fear. I needed to open my heart to all that I was experiencing. Every day, the gift of imagination helped me visualize harmony being restored among the trillions of cells in my body.

It was not an easy time. I would not have consciously chosen cancer as a teacher, but I now appreciate the valuable lessons it offered. Cancer led me to look deeper and to understand that our inherent gifts do indeed have healing power. They can help us heal ourselves, one another, and the world. Accessing them begins with willingness. Gratitude increases their flow.

I hope that Mater's blessings will encourage you to become more aware of your gifts and to help others to see theirs. For are we not all on a healing journey?

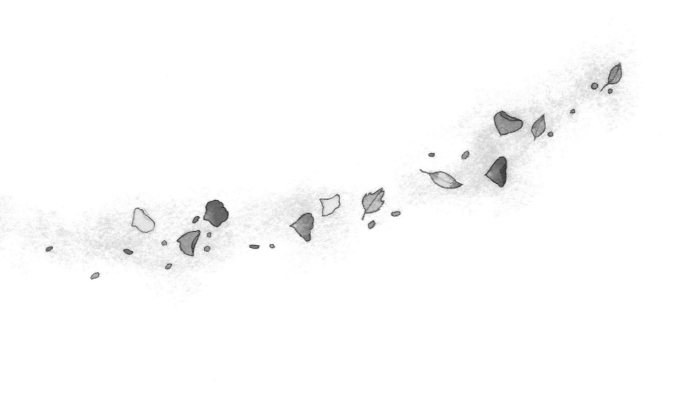

Then your light shall break forth

    like the dawn

and healing spring up quickly.

—ISAIAH 58:8

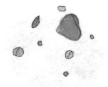

Acknowledgments

There are many people I wish to thank, but I cannot name everyone. I appreciate all who gave help, love, support, and insights during my first book journey throughout the United States, during my healing journey, and on the creative journey toward making this book possible.

On *The Twelve Gifts of Birth* nationwide tour, I encountered thousands of children and adults who helped me better understand the gifts through their responses and their stories. I thank all of you, especially the teachers and therapists who continue to use *The Twelve Gifts of Birth* in your work.

During my cancer crisis, many people helped me rouse the power of my healing place. Again, I can't name everyone but among them are: my husband, Frank; my daughters, Stephanie and Krista; my brother, Keith; and all of my extended family and friends. I thank Krista in particular for the booklet she wrote and illustrated for me. Combining her knowledge as a physician with compassionate understanding and love, she showed cancer cells leaving and my healthy cells having a great celebration. Every time I looked at it, I was filled with hope. I also thank Rev. Kyra Hines Baehr and Unity of Divine Love family. I thank body workers — Kelly, Sandy, Ushi, Divyo, and Melodie as well as Lois and her healing group — who through various forms of healing approaches helped me to allow fear to melt away and to increase harmony, hope, and wholeness. I thank Dr. Jack Cavalcant and Desert Oncology and Dr. Edward Feldman and the Mayo Clinic. Along with excellent medical treatment, both showed me strength, hope, and compassion.

I am grateful for all the sacred places in nature that nourish and help heal us with their beauty. Along with ocean beaches, Red Rock trails, national forests, state parks, wildflower-covered meadows, and rolling green hills, my favorite health promoting places include: Mt. Saint Benedict's Monastery in Erie, PA; Kripalu Center for Yoga and Health in Lenox, MA; the Franciscan Renewal Center in Scottsdale, AZ; and the Chopra Center for Well-Being in Carlsbad, CA.

Assisting with this book and the overall *Twelve Gifts* message, I thank Ling Lucas, my agent; all my friends at HarperCollins, including Cathy Hemming, Megan Newman, Kathryn Huck, Leah Carlson-Stanisic, Shelby Meizlik, Kate Stark, Diane Burrowes, Stephen Hanselman, Mary Ellen Curley, Donna Ruvituso, Karen Lumley, and Jessica Chin; illustrator Alexis Seabrook; book designer Deborah Kerner; and for photo tinting, Richard Waxberg and Todd McQueen. I thank all who listened to early versions of *The Twelve Gifts for Healing* and offered suggestions. Among them: Sister Carolyn Gorny-Kopkowski, Anne Attunes Hawes, Nancy Greystone, Susan Kay Wyatt, Karla Olsen, Karen Heard, Trish and Paul Howey, Gayle Kump, Linda Hanniford, Marilyn Greco, Linda Simon, Tina Higgins, Margaret Woodlief, Mary Lu Jordan-Elliot, and Marianne Keis. I thank Karen Heard also for the preliminary design and cover design.

I thank booksellers and retailers who carry *The Twelve Gifts* books. I thank readers who, when touched by them, share *The Twelve Gifts* message with others.

Finally, but first and above all, I thank the One from whom all gifts flow.

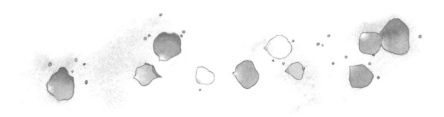

To learn more about

The Twelve Gifts

or to contact Charlene Costanzo

please visit

www.TheTwelveGifts.com

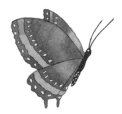